TEENS DEALING WITH
MENTAL ILLNESS

by Philip Wolny

BrightPoint Press

San Diego, CA

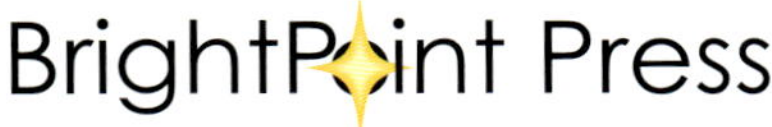

Content Consultant: Lindsey Weiler, PhD, Associate Professor of Family Social Science, University of Minnesota

LIBRARY OF CONGRESS CATALOGING-IN-PUBLICATION DATA

Names: Wolny, Philip, author.
Title: Teens dealing with mental illness / by Philip Wolny.
Description: San Diego, CA: BrightPoint Press, [2025] | Series: Teens dealing with adversity | Includes bibliographical references and index. | Audience: Grades 7-9
Identifiers: LCCN 2024004139 (print) | LCCN 2024004140 (eBook) | ISBN 9781678208905 (hardcover) | ISBN 9781678208912 (eBook)
Subjects: LCSH: Mentally ill teenagers--Juvenile literature. | Teenagers--Mental health--Juvenile literature. | Mental illness--Juvenile literature.
Classification: LCC RJ503 .W65 2025 (print) | LCC RJ503 (eBook) | DDC 616.8900835--dc23/eng/20240227
LC record available at https://lccn.loc.gov/2024004139
LC eBook record available at https://lccn.loc.gov/2024004140

CONTENTS

AT A GLANCE

- Emotions and thoughts can be intense during the teen years.

- Situational depression and anxiety are normal. Depression, anxiety, and other issues that stick around can be signs of mental illness.

- Genetics, someone's environment, trauma, and other factors can lead to symptoms of a mental health disorder.

- Teens may struggle privately with their mental health. Mental illness can lead to serious symptoms such as considering suicide.

- Teens with obsessive-compulsive disorder (OCD) and other anxiety disorders might isolate from friends and family and fixate on certain behaviors and routines.

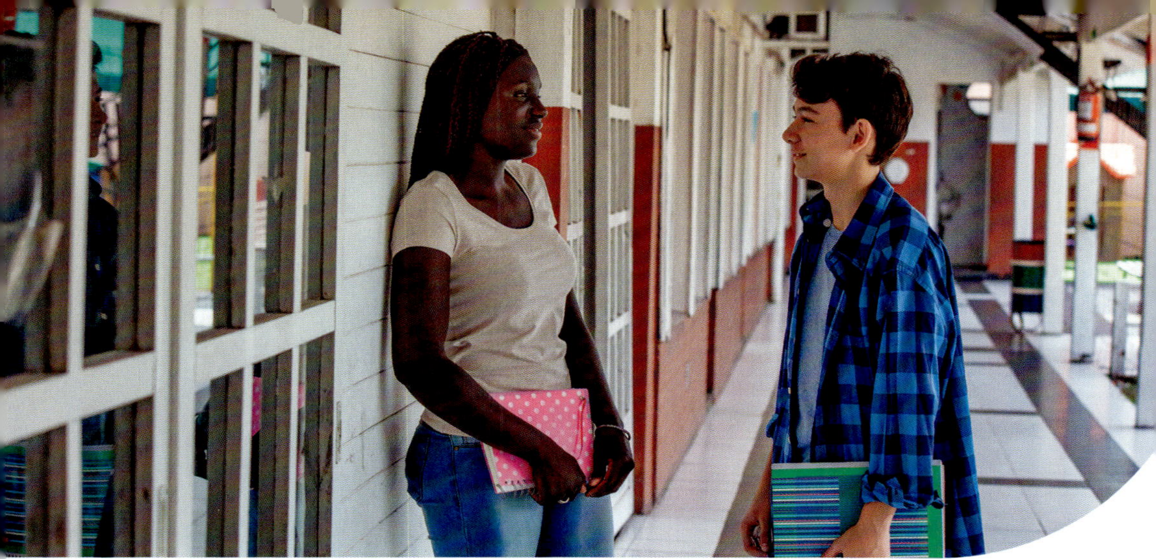

- Therapy allows a patient to talk about their mental health issues. Therapists teach patients to practice special methods to reduce stress and other symptoms of their conditions.

- Self-care can help teens cope with their mental health struggles. Creative outlets and other pursuits are some ways that teens cope with their mental health issues.

- Prescription medications can also help teens cope with their symptoms.

- Building supportive relationships with others can help teens manage their mental health well-being.

SPEAKING UP

In the summer of 2022, a friend asked 17-year-old Yanie to speak at a public forum. At first, the teenager from East Orange, New Jersey, said no. The event was a public discussion about mental illness. Yanie was scared about opening up.

Yanie listened to the other students' stories. Some of the teens came from low-income homes. They had seen gun violence. Some coped by overeating.

Speaking up about mental health can help people connect with each other.

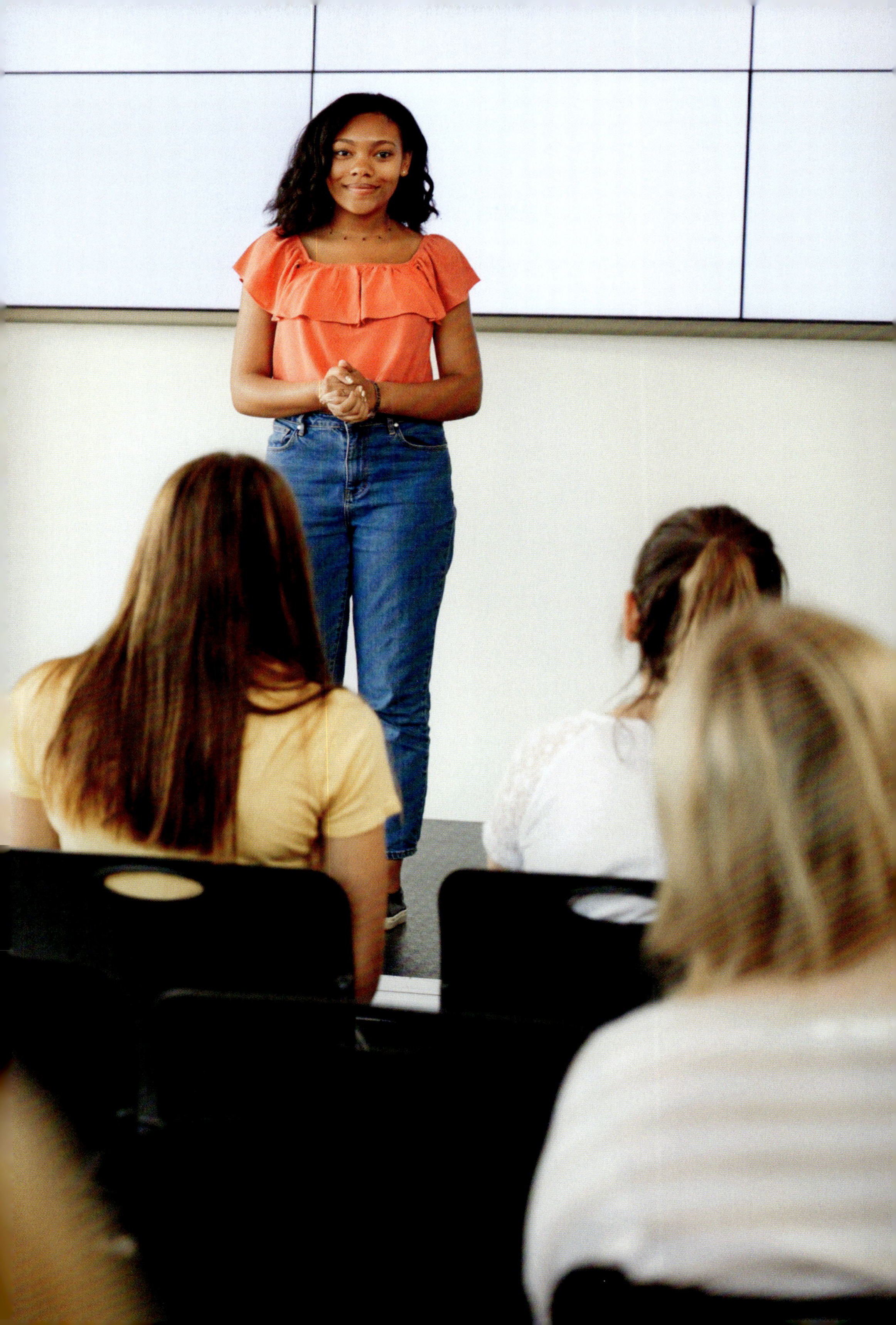

Others engaged in self-harm, such as cutting. Some had even been hospitalized.

Yanie found the courage to speak. She shared that she began showing self-harm behavior at 9 years old. She thought about killing herself. Sometimes she was sad. Other times she felt rage. Her anger was a way of expressing her sadness. She had fights with classmates and was sent to an alternative school.

The COVID-19 pandemic started in 2020. Yanie's mother worked long hours as a nurse. Yanie cared for her two younger brothers during the day. She felt trapped and fell into a deep depression. She barely ate or left her room.

Yanie found an online after-school program. Part of the program taught teens

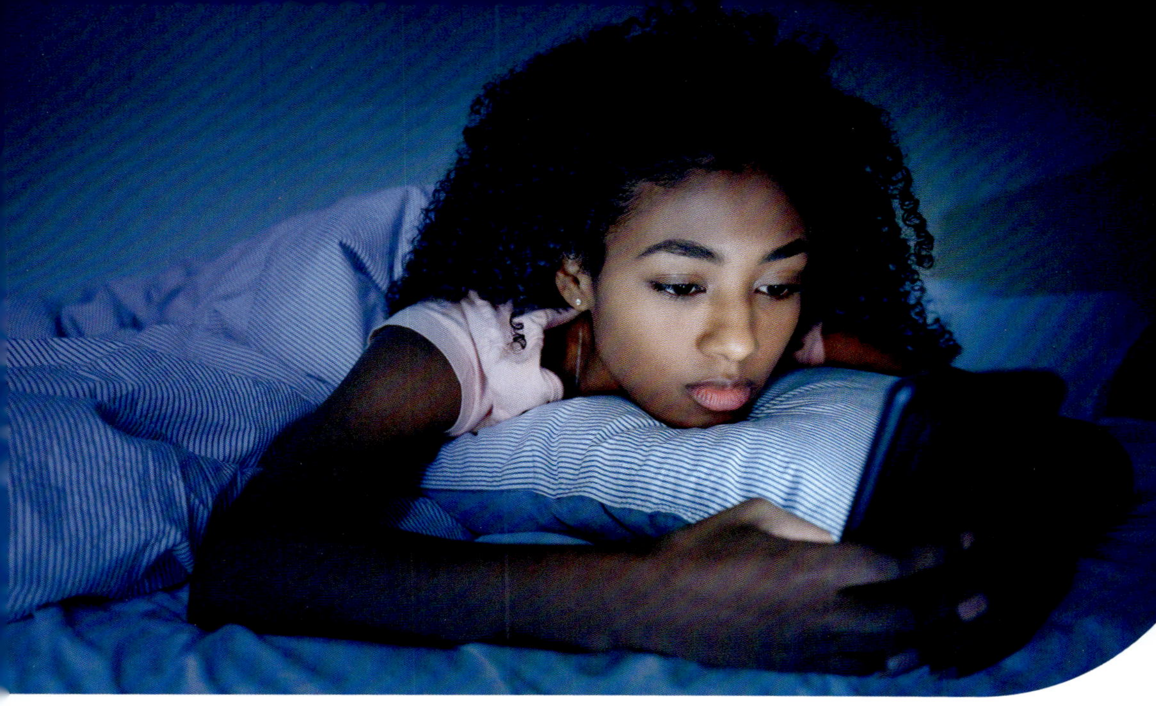

how to deal with their emotions. Yanie met with a social worker named Jamila Davis. She encouraged Yanie to speak at the forum. Yanie hoped her story could help break the **stigma**. Other students said they related to her story. Yanie didn't feel alone in her experience. Yanie's story is just one of millions. Teens living with a mental illness come from all backgrounds. When people speak up, they show they are not alone.

CHAPTER ONE

FEELING INTENSE EMOTIONS

Everyone has bad days. For teenagers, some days are worse than others. Teens face pressure to juggle family, sports, school, and a social life.

A teenager's body and mind go through many changes as they grow. It can be confusing and stressful. Daily stresses are common. Some teens may experience difficult feelings such as sadness or anger more often than their classmates.

Teens face a lot of pressure to succeed in school.

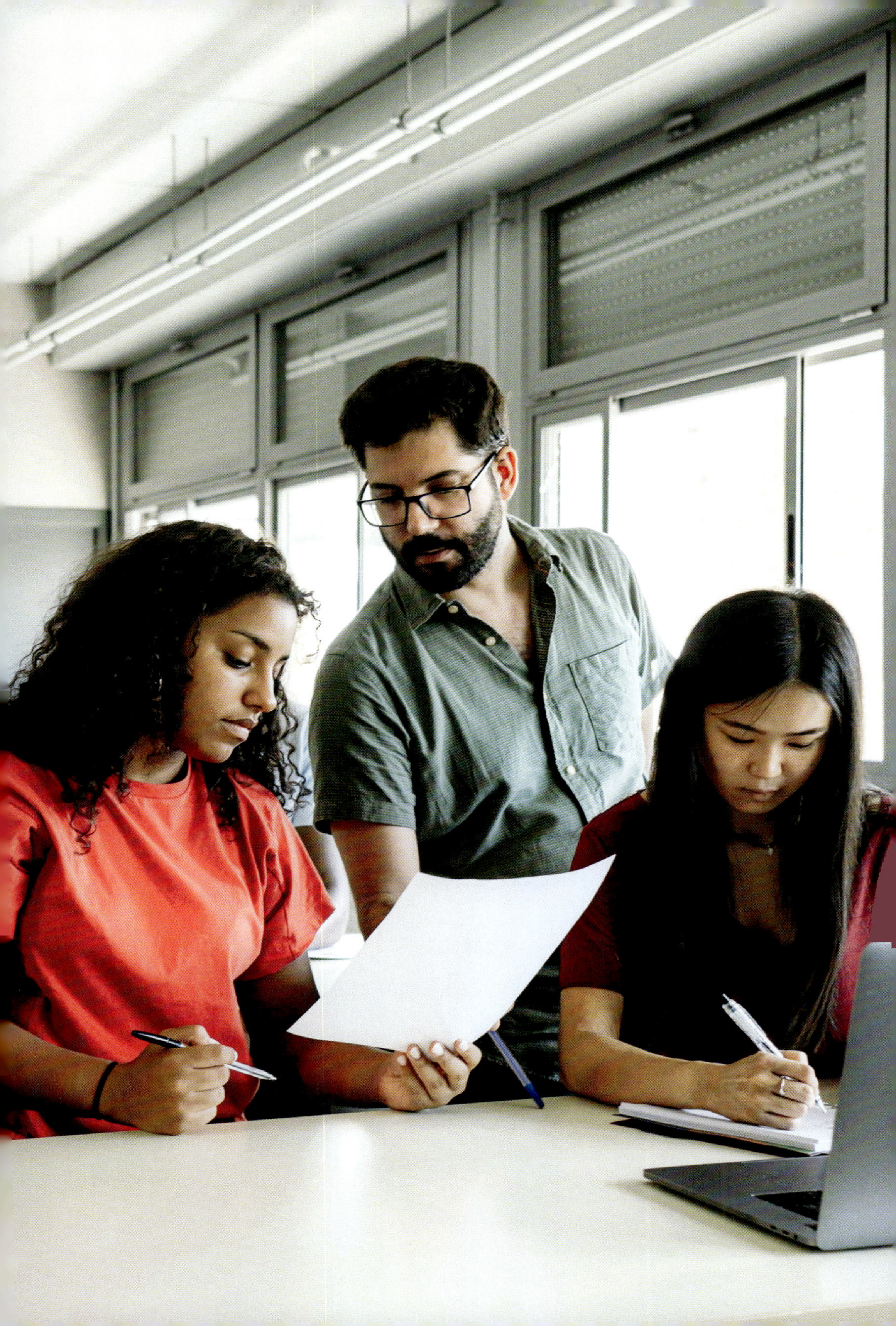

WHAT IS MENTAL ILLNESS?

Emotions are a part of growing up. Moving to a new area can cause anxiety. The first day of school can be stressful. Teens worry about making friends or doing well in classes. The death of a family member or friend might make them feel depressed.

Situational depression or anxiety can occur after a recent tragedy.

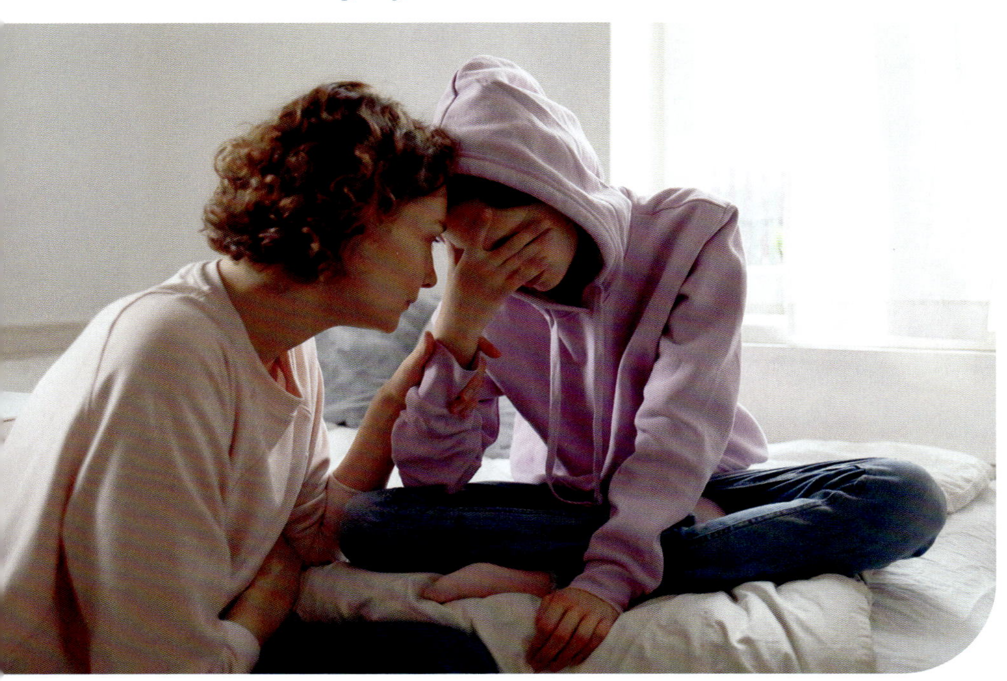

These feelings of anxiety or depression
are situational.

Sometimes, intense feelings stick around.
There may not seem to be any reason for
them. These feelings might be a sign of
mental illness.

The American Psychiatric Association
(APA) defines mental illnesses as "health
conditions involving changes in emotion,
thinking, or behavior, or a combination of
these." Trouble controlling one's emotions
and behavior may be a sign of mental
illness. So are negative or irrational thoughts
that affect daily life.

SIGNS OF MENTAL ILLNESS

There are many warning signs of mental
illness. One is a person losing interest in

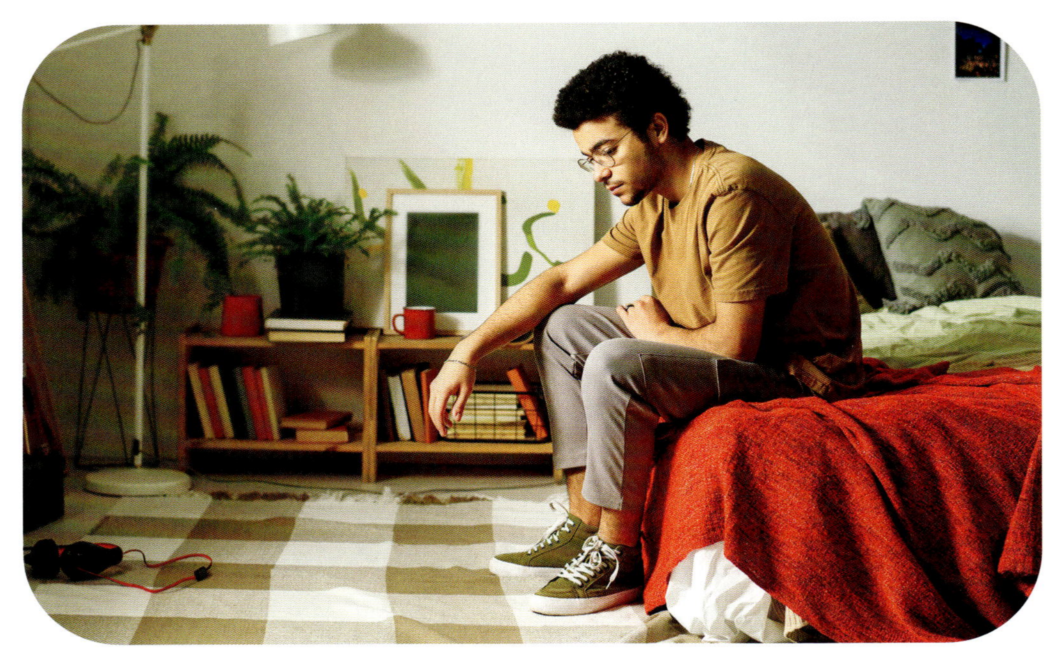

If someone begins to lose interest in hobbies they once enjoyed, it may be a sign that they are struggling with their mental health.

things they used to enjoy. This might include sports or hobbies. Another sign is low energy. A teen might sleep more than usual or sleep late.

Mental illness can affect a teen's diet and activity. They may have a sudden loss of appetite. Another teen might overeat or binge eat. Some teens may cope by exercising or dieting too much.

Destructive and risky behaviors are also warning signs of mental illness. A common symptom is self-harm, such as cutting. Other people might turn to alcohol or other drugs to cope with deeper issues.

A serious sign of mental illness is having thoughts of suicide. Some teens may speak or write about suicide. Other warning signs can sometimes go unnoticed. These signs may include giving away belongings, sudden shifts in mood, or withdrawing from family and friends.

ANXIETY AND DEPRESSION

Many teens have anxiety. The US Department of Health and Human Services says that about 32 percent of 13- to 18-year-olds experience anxiety.

Generalized anxiety disorder shows itself as extreme worry and anxiety that is hard to manage. Teens suffering from anxiety may fear going to school or leaving the house.

Social anxiety is an intense fear of being around other people. It is more serious than general shyness. The thought of speaking to others may cause panic attacks.

Another common mental disorder is depression. Some people confuse depression with sadness. Regular sadness will eventually pass. Major depressive disorder may not go away without treatment. Depression affects how someone feels, thinks, and acts.

In 2023, about 11.5 percent of youth reported experiencing major depression. Over 16 percent of 12- to 17-year-olds had

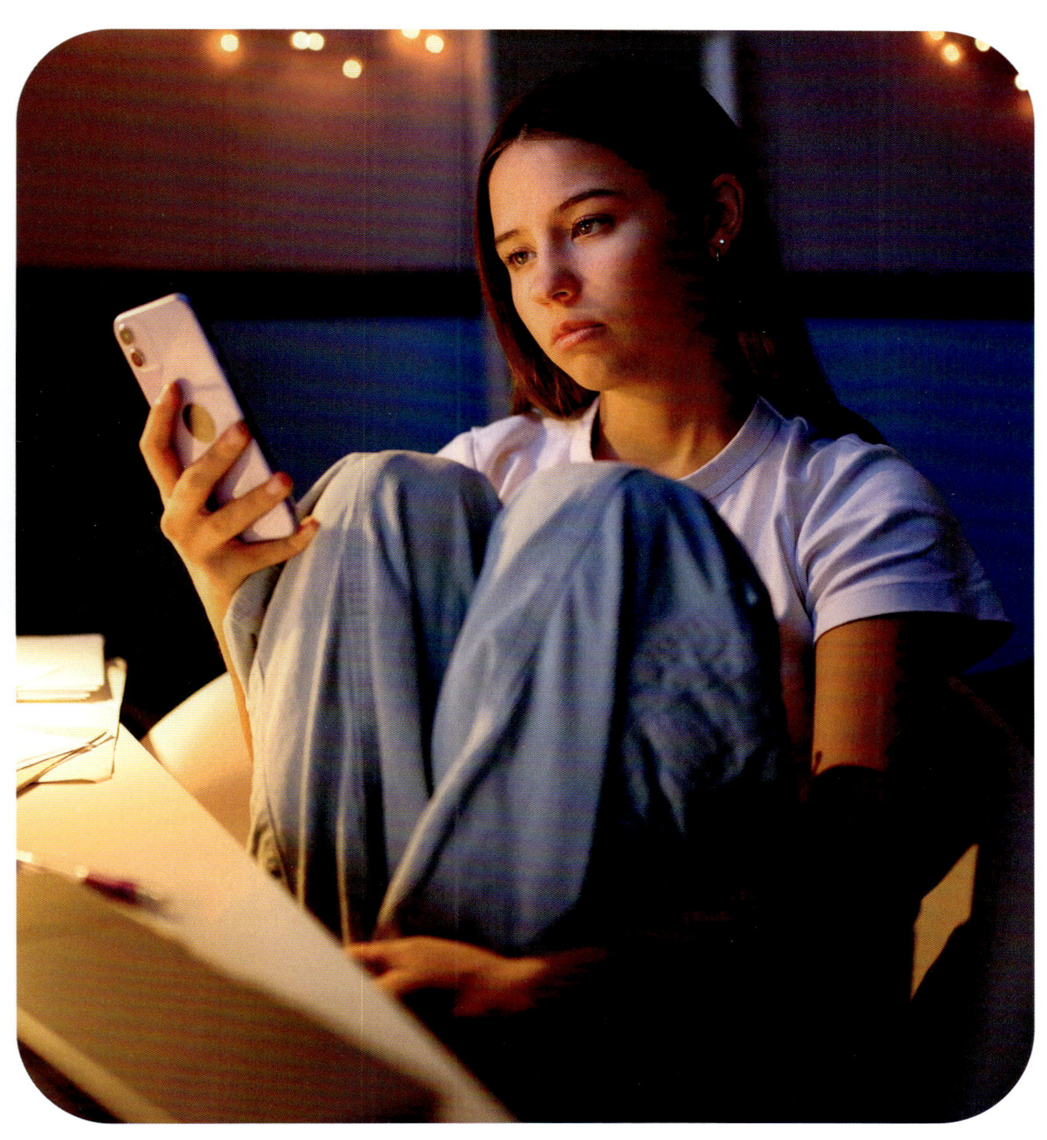

Some people may avoid going out with friends due to intense social anxiety.

at least one major depressive episode

in 2023. Such an episode is a period of

depression lasting at least 2 weeks.

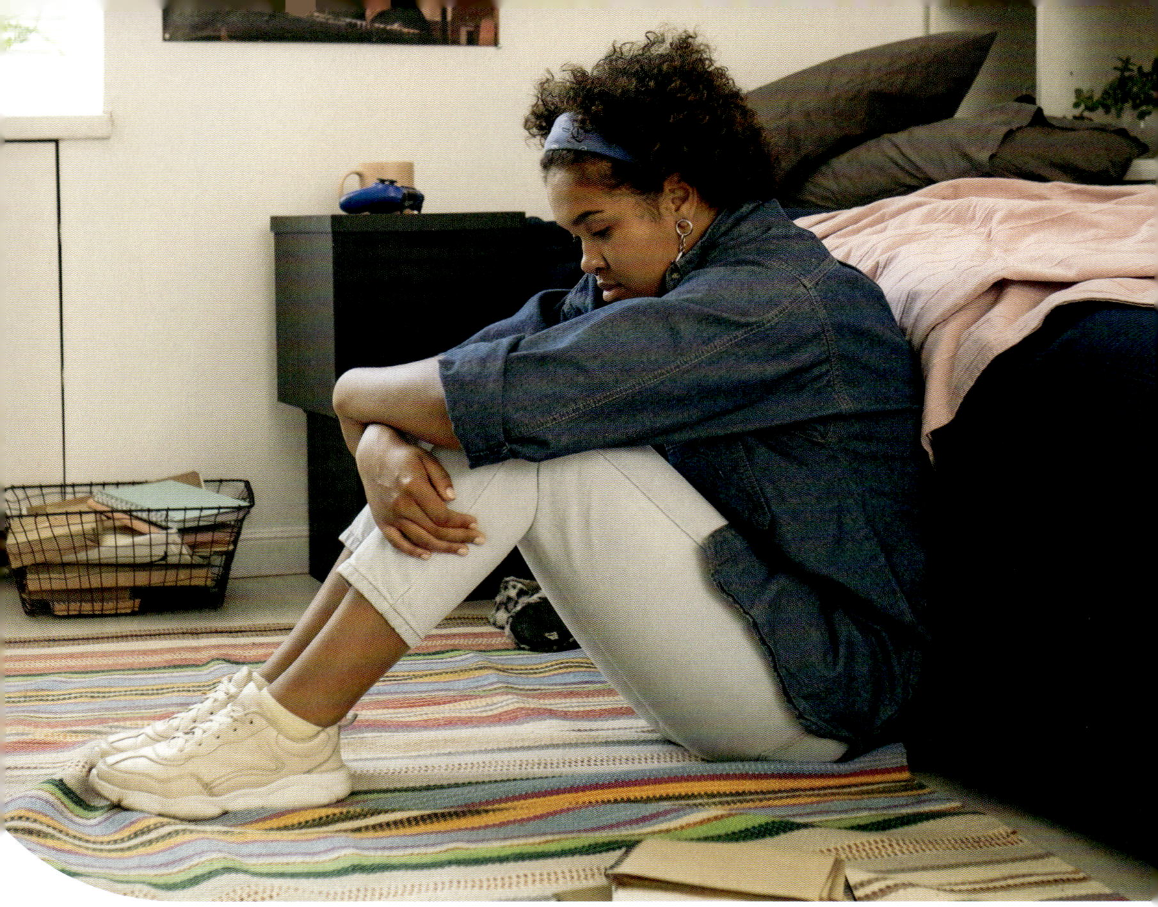

Withdrawing from friends and family may be a sign that someone is depressed.

Dr. Craig Sawchuk of the Mayo Clinic explains some of the feelings that depression brings. He says,

"Emotionally, you may feel sad or down or irritable . . . the body really slows down. You feel tired. Your sleep is often disrupted. It's really hard to

get yourself motivated. Your thinking also changes. It can just be hard to concentrate. Your thoughts tend to be much more negative. You can be really hard on yourself, feel hopeless and helpless about things."[1]

Someone with a mental illness may have one or more conditions or disorders. They may have several symptoms that require treatment. Many people are **diagnosed** with both depression and anxiety.

OTHER KINDS OF MENTAL ILLNESS

Mental illnesses often affect how teens view themselves. About 3 percent of 13- to 18-year-olds experience eating disorders. People with anorexia have a restrictive diet. Those with bulimia might eat a lot of food at once, then force themselves to vomit. This becomes an unhealthy cycle of binging and **purging**.

Obsessive-compulsive disorder (OCD) is another issue some young people face. About 1 in 200 young people have OCD. It causes actions or thoughts that someone feels they cannot control. Some people may wash their hands dozens of times per day. They repeat actions over and over. They may become obsessed with having things in their room arranged a certain way. If they don't follow these behaviors, they experience extreme anxiety and distress.

People with bipolar disorder (BD) will experience big mood swings over time. About 2.9 percent of US teens have BD. Someone might be very depressed for a few weeks or months. Then they experience emotional highs known as **manic** episodes. They may have lots of sudden energy. They can also get easily irritated. These changes in moods can affect sleeping patterns and judgment. A bipolar teen may act in **impulsive** ways. They may

Many teens have issues with their self-image. This can lead to eating disorders.

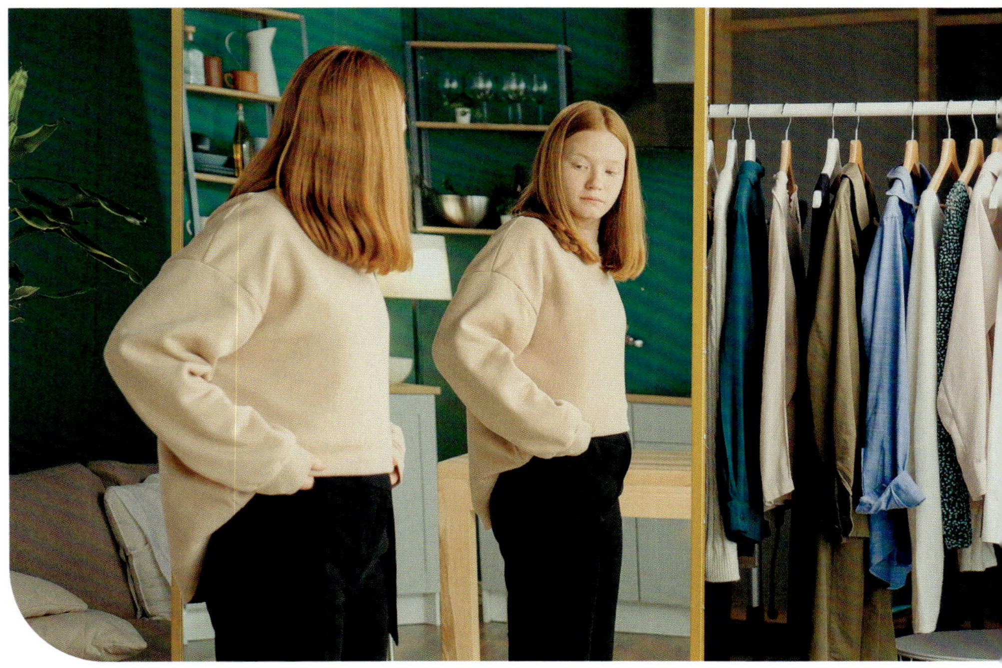

behave recklessly and put themselves in dangerous situations.

Another type of mental disorder is attention-deficit/**hyperactivity** disorder (ADHD). About 9 percent of 13- to 18-year-olds experience it. People with ADHD find it very hard to concentrate on daily tasks. This may happen while taking a test or having a conversation with someone.

It can be hard for teens with ADHD to focus in class.

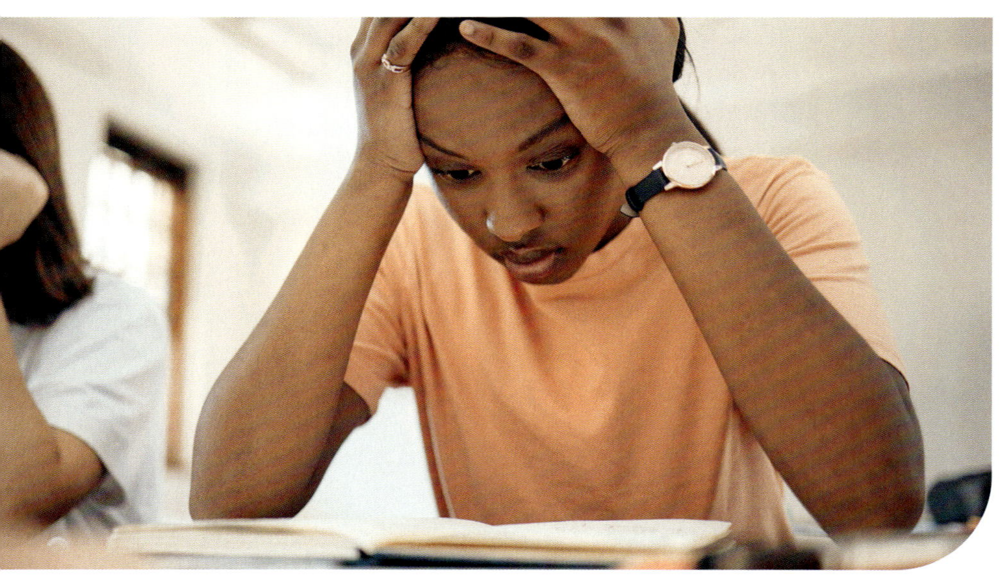

Hyperactivity is a common symptom. They
might do things without thinking about them
first. These symptoms can make it hard for
teens to focus in school.

WHERE DO MENTAL ILLNESSES COME FROM?

The National Institutes of Health say that
several factors affect teen mental health.
Genes may play a role. A family history
of mental health issues can mean a
higher risk for certain disorders. Bipolar
disorder, ADHD, major depression, and
schizophrenia are all believed to be tied to
genetic history.

Chemicals in the brain help control
moods, emotions, and behavior. An
imbalance in brain chemicals can disrupt

mental health. Many drugs prescribed
to help those with mental illnesses help
balance out these substances in the brain.

Someone's personal experiences and
upbringing can also negatively affect their
mental health. A person experiencing
poverty may have anxiety more often than
others. Poor relationships with family can
seriously affect teens as well.

Children can experience trauma.
Mental health professionals sometimes

Schizophrenia

Schizophrenia affects how someone experiences
reality. Hallucinations and strange thoughts
such as **delusions** are common. Less than
.04 percent of children are estimated to
develop schizophrenia.

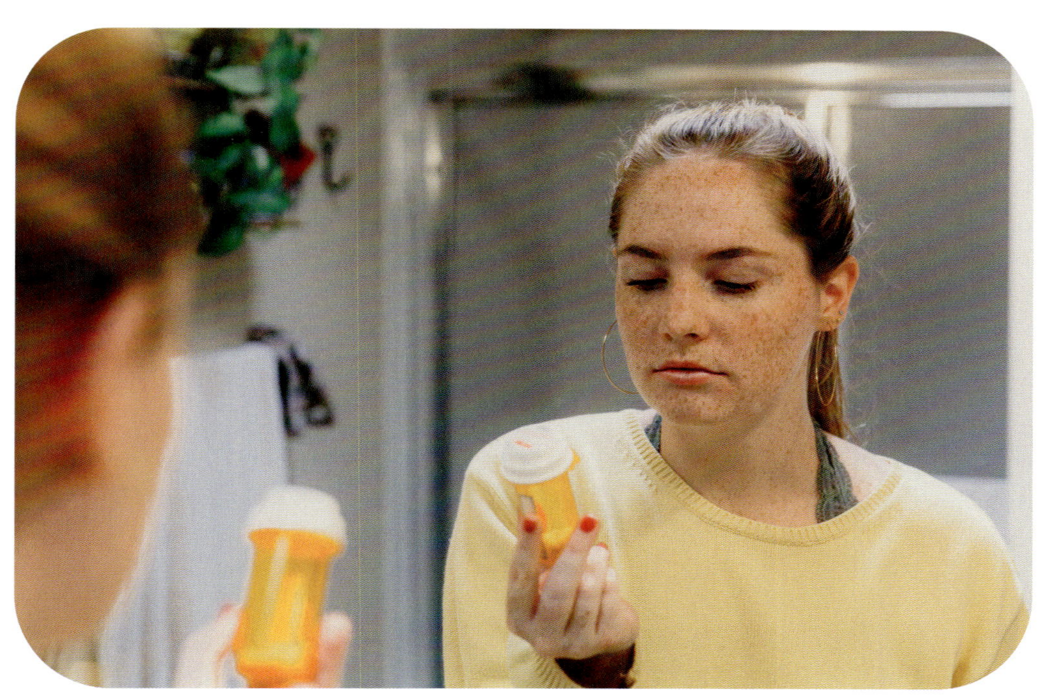

Psychiatrists may prescribe medication to help people manage mental illness symptoms.

call such events adverse childhood experiences. Neglect and physical abuse can affect mental health as well. Some children are bullied or socially isolated. Racism, homophobia, or other forms of discrimination can also cause depression and anxiety in teens. Abusing drugs and alcohol negatively affects someone's mental health as well.

CHAPTER TWO

OVERCOMING HURDLES

It can feel hard to speak up about struggling with mental illness. Speaking up is the first step in feeling less alone. Finding people to talk to can help make the process less scary.

The next step is finding a diagnosis. Once a diagnosis is made, figuring out the best treatment can be possible. It is never too late to speak up and find help.

Finding the courage to talk about mental health issues can be difficult at first.

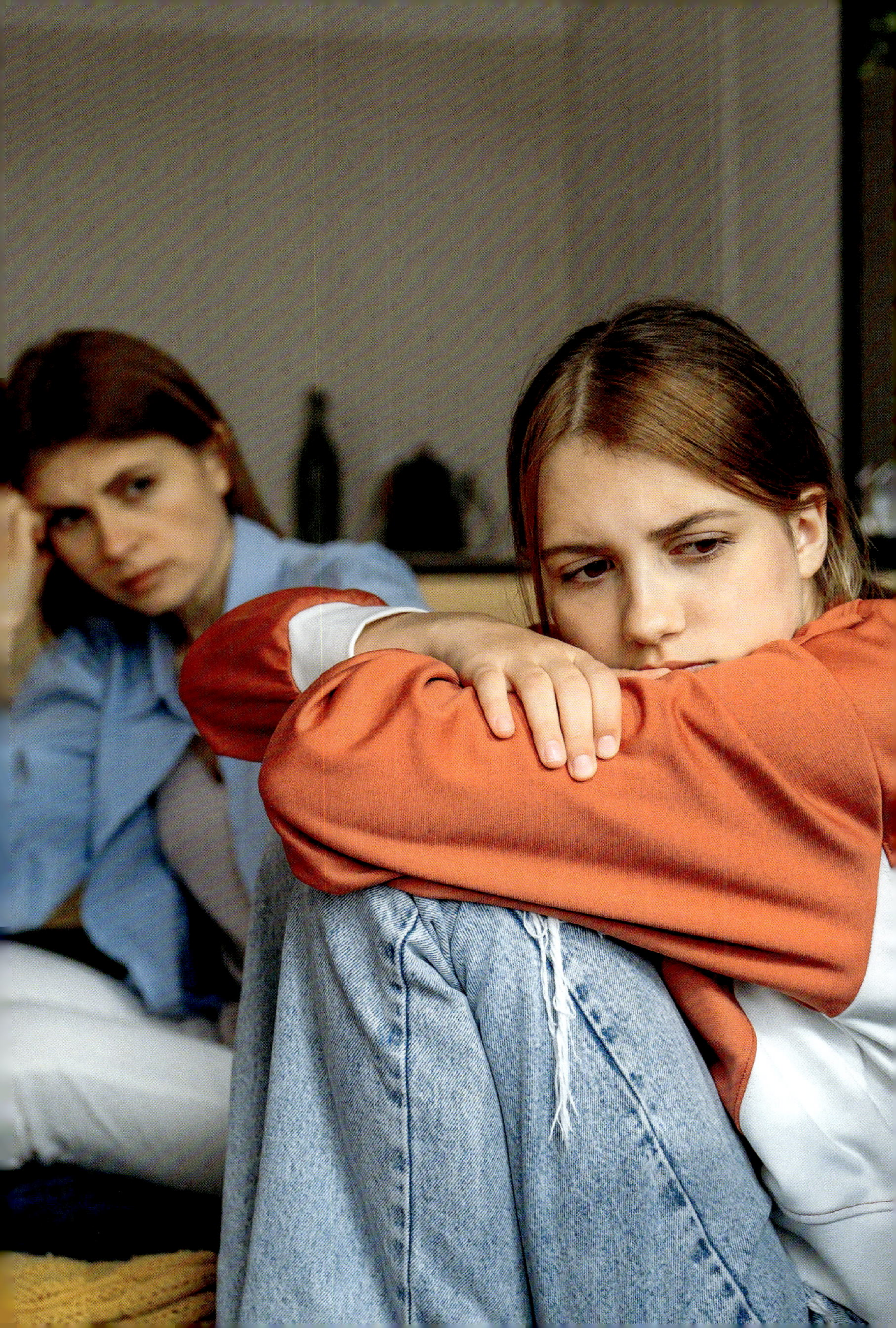

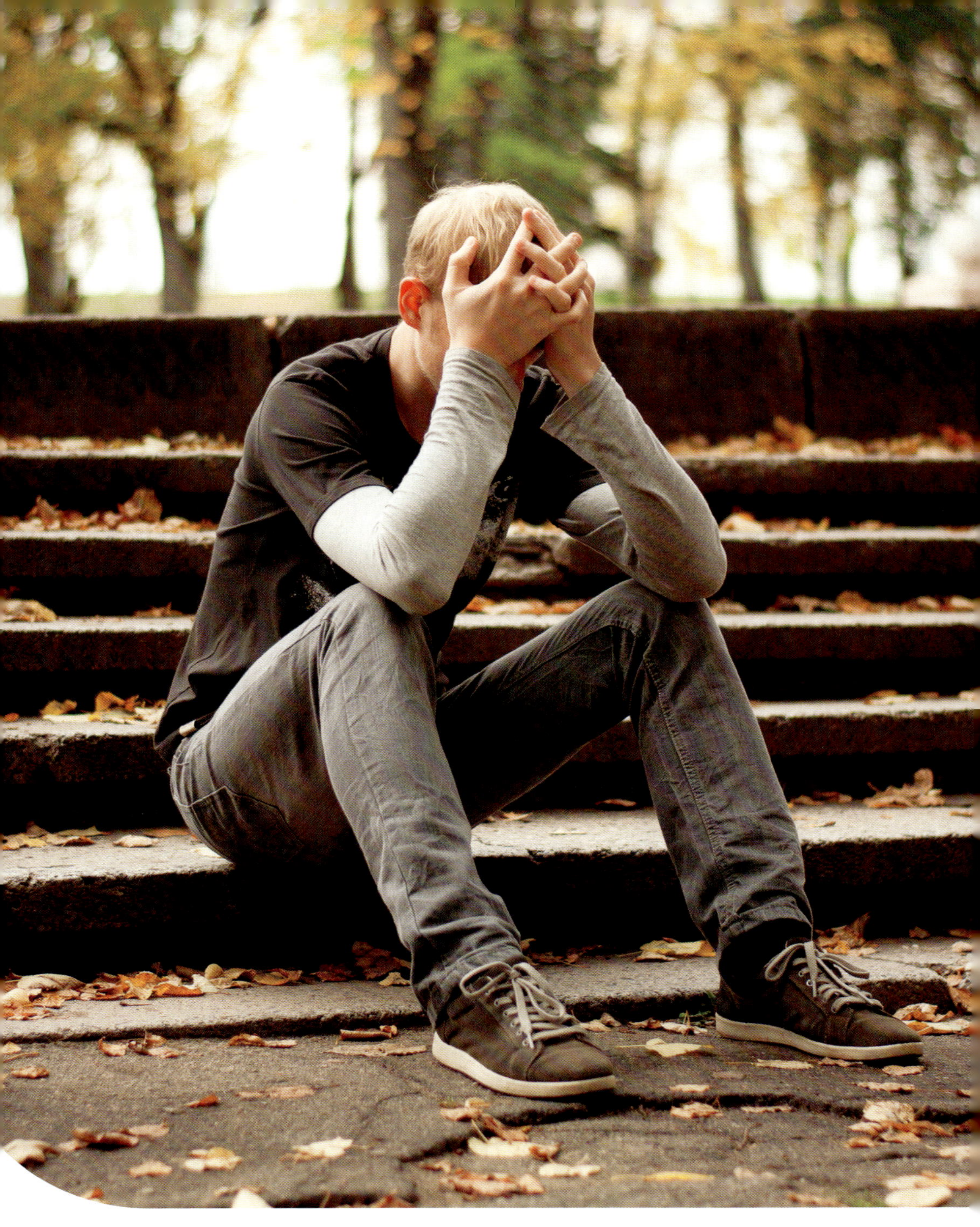

The pressure to succeed can cause teens to feel overwhelmed.

A PRIVATE STRUGGLE

Carson was a teenager living near Green Bay, Wisconsin. He felt a lot of pressure to do well in academics and sports. This pressure made him feel as if he was never good enough. He hid his struggles. One morning, his mother heard a gunshot. Carson's family found him in the family garage. He had shot himself in the face, but survived.

The pressure Carson felt gave him severe anxiety and depression. He talked to ABC News about his depression in 2021. "I describe it as like falling into a black hole," Carson explained. "It's quick, unexpected, scary and dark. It went to the point where I thought the only way I was going to get rid of those feelings was to try and take my own life."[2]

His mental illness had worsened because he felt he had no way to express his emotions. He finally got the help he needed. He started going to therapy. Carson realized talking about his experience could help others. Carson had many surgeries after his suicide attempt. Doctors worked to reconstruct his face.

Carson started a TikTok account to share his story. One of his posts got thousands of responses. Carson's TikTok account helped other teens deal with their suicidal feelings. He and his mother have also spoken with lawmakers about improving teen mental health services.

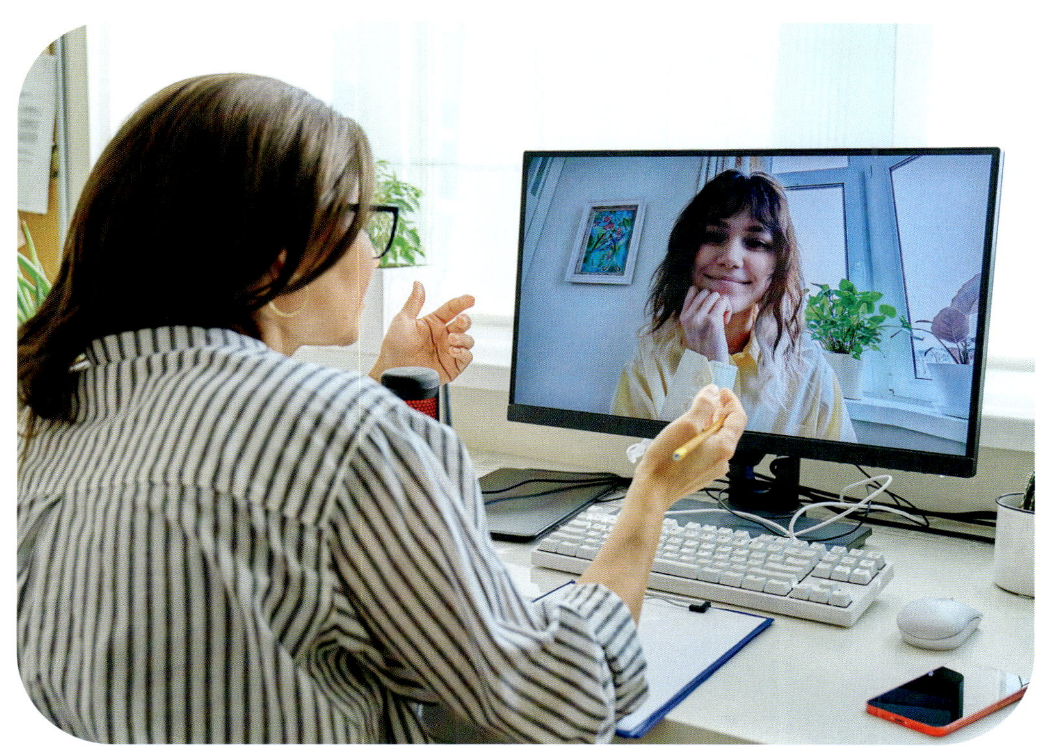

Telehealth can make therapy more accessible for patients.

Carson wants states to expand telehealth therapy. Instead of having to meet in person, Carson can meet from home via video call. He knows there are teens who are too anxious to make in-person appointments. They might feel more comfortable seeking therapy from home.

LOSING CONTROL

The Child Mind Institute is a clinic that helps teens and young adults with mental health issues. Dr. Jerry Bubrick treated 13-year-old Ben from New York. Bubrick interviewed

Therapists can help by providing a diagnosis.

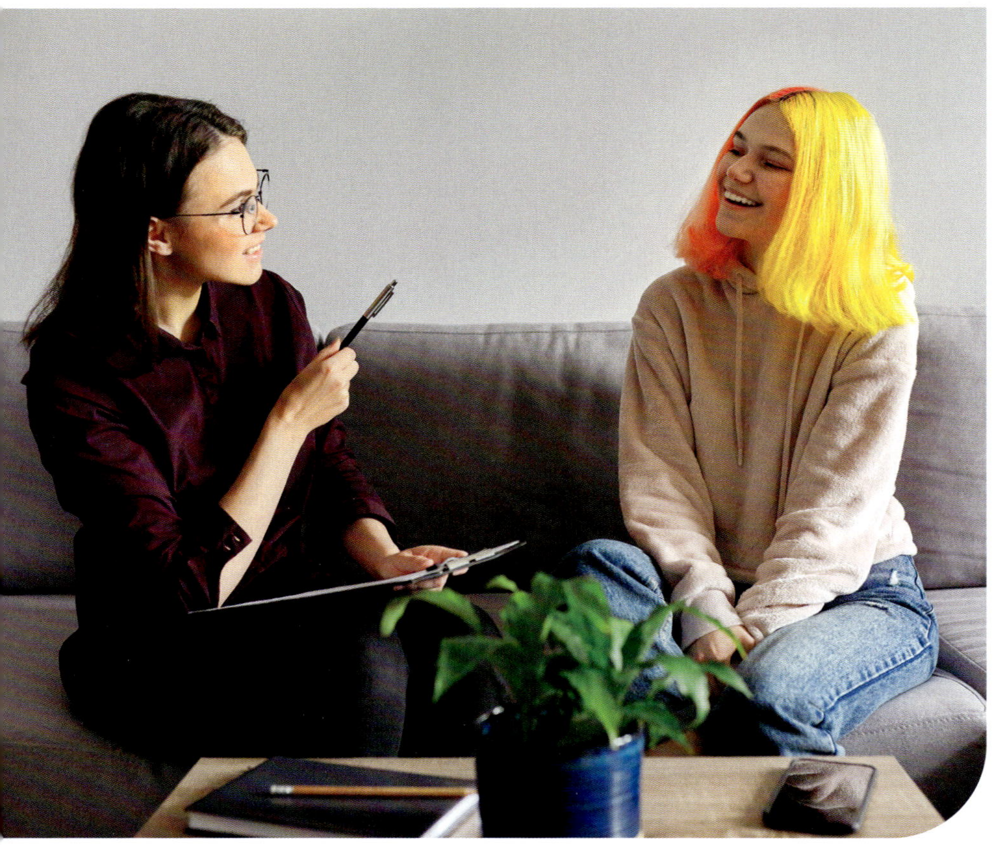

Ben on the Child Mind Institute website about Ben's OCD diagnosis.

Ben was around 6 or 7 years old when he started checking behind his bed for robbers. He knew no one could fit back there. But it made him feel better at night.

One day, Ben started obsessing over his parents abandoning him. He imagined them sneaking out while he slept. His parents had to reassure him that they would not leave. Ben even started sleeping on a mattress on their bedroom floor.

A therapist diagnosed Ben with OCD. His weekly therapy seemed to be helping at first. But his OCD grew more severe. Ben said, "I was touching things, thinking 'Oh, if I touch this, Mom and Dad won't leave, it will be okay.'"[3]

His habits worsened in the summer after seventh grade. Ben attended a tennis camp and played on a baseball team. He would panic about being away from his parents. When school started, Ben would call his parents from the school therapist's office.

Ben visited a psychiatrist. The psychiatrist prescribed him Zoloft. This is a drug that helps with OCD, depression, anxiety, and other issues. He also took Xanax. It is used to ease panic attacks and anxiety. It took days for Ben to get used to the medications. He felt calmer, but his OCD seemed even worse. Ben could not even leave his room. The idea of attending school was unbearable.

Finally, Ben's mother found Dr. Bubrick. Bubrick used exposure therapy for

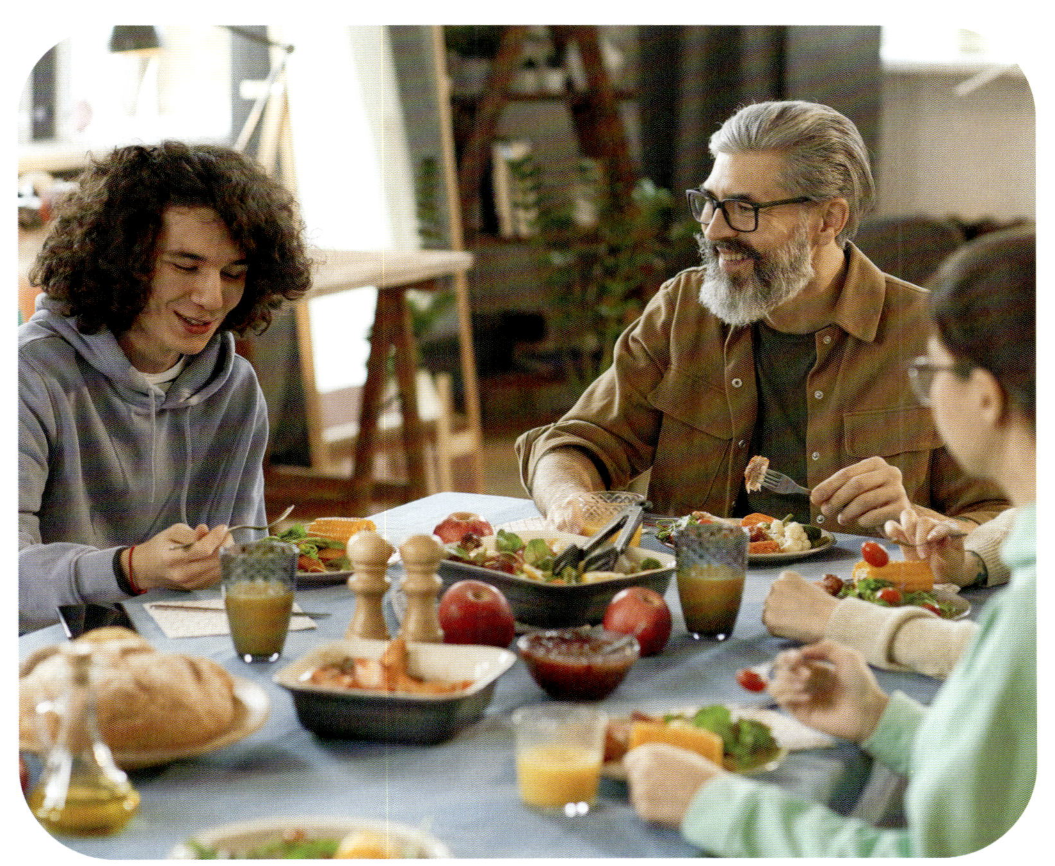

Families can be a part of the healing process at home.

Ben's OCD. He exposed Ben to things he feared twice a week. At home, his parents helped him with his exposures as well.

When his parents went to the grocery store, Ben would practice dealing with his anxiety. Over time, they could stay out longer. The more he practiced his exposures, the better he felt. Eventually, he was able to be alone for long periods of time.

RETHINKING MENTAL ILLNESS

Christine Marie was happy and outgoing. She was popular, a good student, and an athlete. She started feeling anxiety

Mental Health During the COVID-19 Pandemic

In 2020, the COVID-19 pandemic forced many schools to close. Dr. Marcie Billings of the Mayo Clinic pointed out that for teens, "That's their time to start to be independent and start to exert some control over their own lives. And that was taken away in a way that we had never experienced before."[4]

in elementary school. The anxiety got worse when she turned 12 years old. She also developed depression. She hid her feelings to get by. She wanted to seem normal. In seventh grade, Christine Marie's parents noticed her struggling and got her professional help. However, her problems continued to get worse.

Christine Marie experienced **psychosis** brought on by her BD diagnosis. She started hallucinating. Christine Marie lost all of her friends. She felt hopeless and fed up. She was tired of being known as mentally ill. Christine Marie and her mom came up with a new term, Brain XP. This was short for "brain eXPanded." Using the term Brain XP gave the teen a positive way to think about herself.

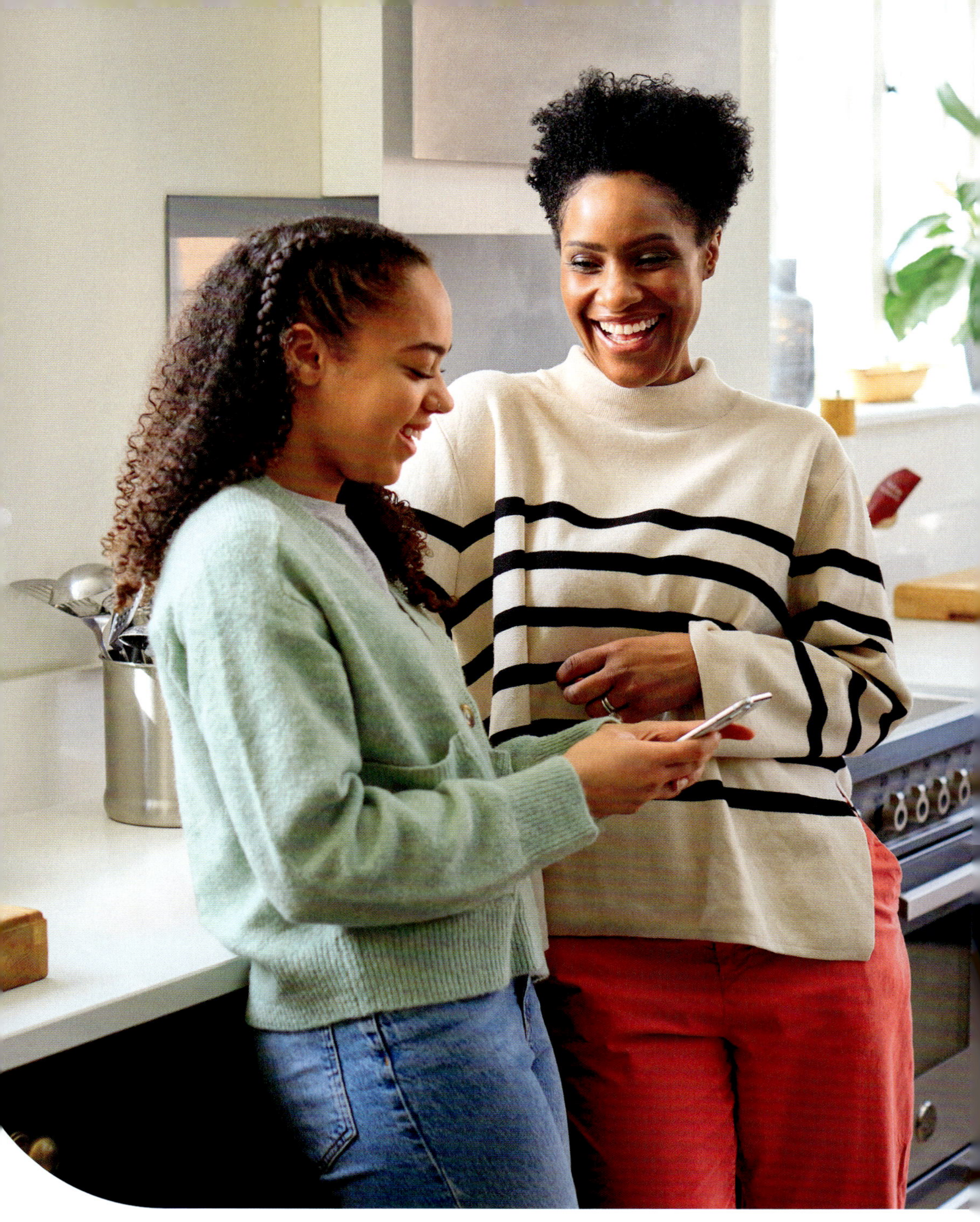

Social media can be used as a tool to help teens feel connected and heard.

Christine Marie decided to write a book about her personal story. She included steps she took to cope with her illness. One tool she used was songwriting. The book expanded into a website and other projects.

Today, Christine Marie uses social media to spread awareness about mental health. The Brain XP Project also educates and trains young people to help friends in need. The National Alliance on Mental Illness (NAMI) awarded Christine Marie with the 2019 Youth Advocate of the Year Award.

LIVING WITH MENTAL ILLNESS

Teens cope with mental disorders in many ways. Each young person's path toward mental wellness is a personal one. Therapy, medication, or other techniques can all help teens cope.

Most mental illnesses do not have a cure. Healing does not work the way it does for physical issues like a broken arm. But people can find helpful ways to manage and minimize their symptoms.

There are many ways for teens to cope with their mental illness.

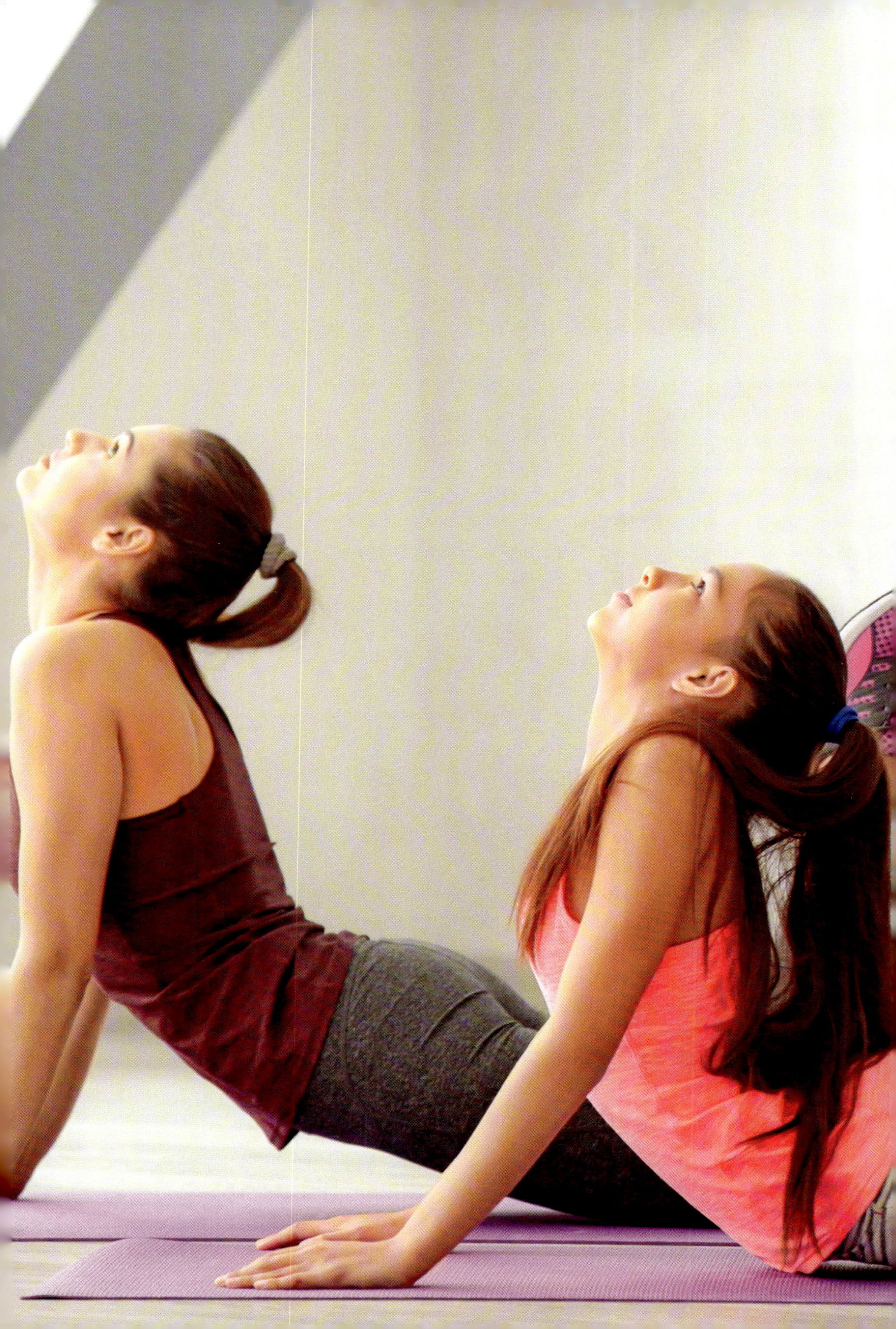

TALKING IT THROUGH

A first step in treating mental illness is finding someone to talk to and getting a diagnosis. Therapists and psychologists are two kinds of professionals who help with mental health issues. One of their main healing tools is psychotherapy, also known as talk therapy. School counselors and social workers can also help.

Different kinds of therapy work for different patients and situations. Many patients see a therapist once a week. Other people might need more frequent sessions when they are going through a rough time. Their caregiver might plan out a mix of individual and group therapy sessions.

Tobias J. Atkins told his story to the Anxiety & Depression Association

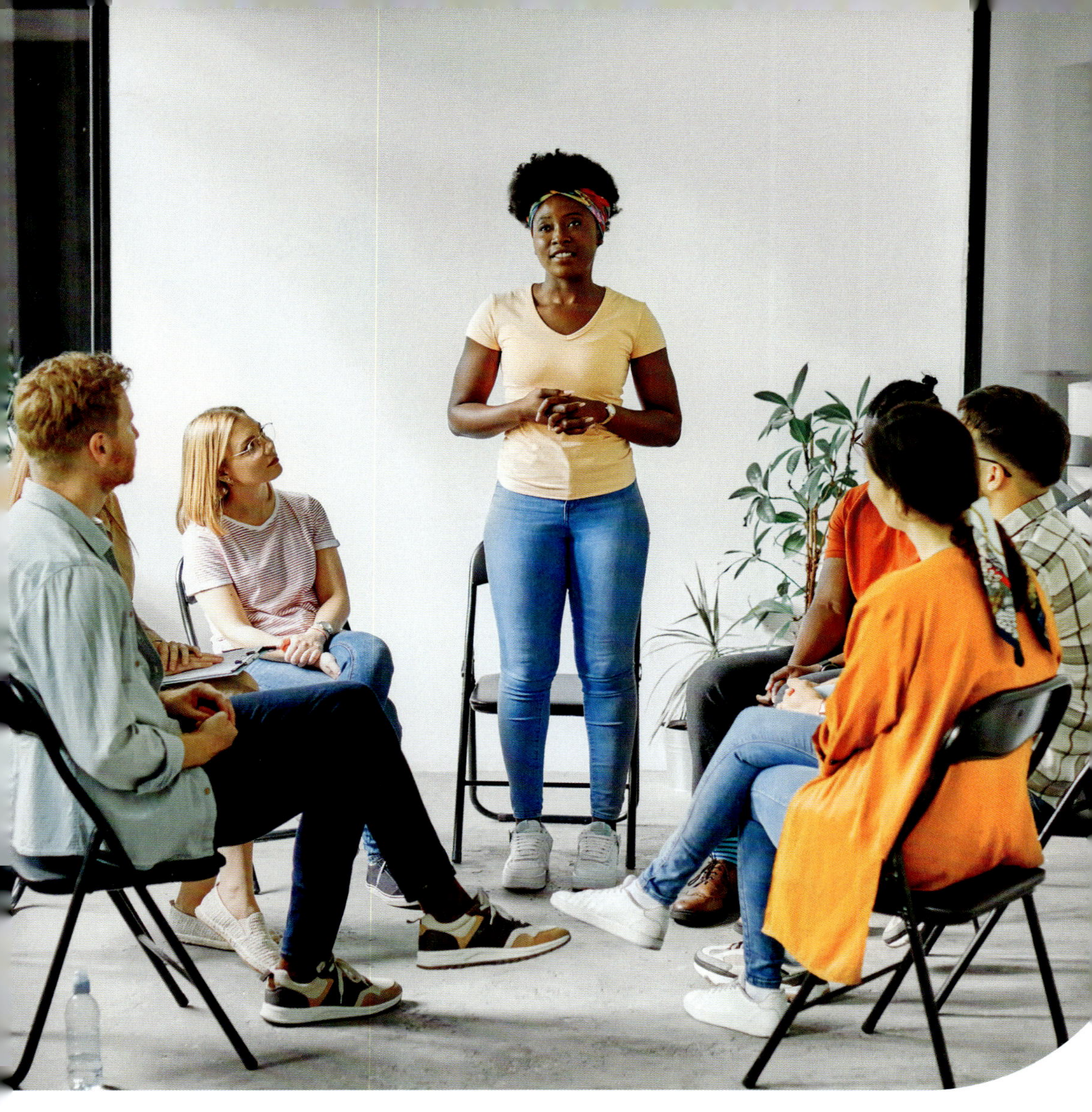

Group therapy gives patients an opportunity to meet with other people who may be struggling with similar issues.

of America (ADAA). Atkins suffered

throughout childhood with social anxiety,

generalized anxiety, depression, and OCD.

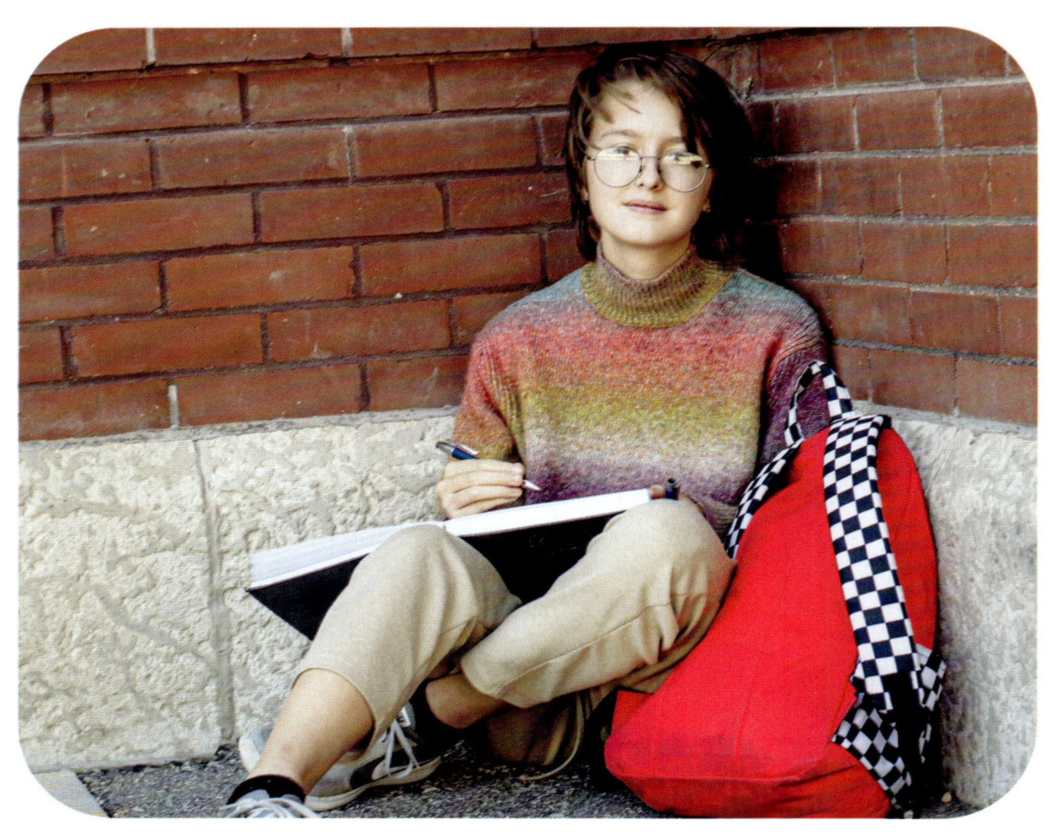

Social anxiety may prevent teens from wanting to socialize with their peers.

His problems continued into adulthood. Atkins said,

> *"I found it difficult to relax and be myself around people, even with friends that I have known for years. . . . I believed I was born shy, and there was nothing I could do to fix it, so I*

didn't even try. . . . I was raised to believe it was weak to talk about feelings. . . . I have since come to realize that admitting you need help and talking about your feelings is one of the bravest things you can do."[5]

Atkins's life changed after he went to a psychologist. He learned to stop thinking of himself negatively. He learned self-acceptance. He did not have to

Cognitive Behavioral Therapy (CBT)

Cognitive Behavioral Therapy (CBT) is a common type of talk therapy. Patients are shown how to change their self-image. Therapists help them fight negative and unhelpful ways of thinking. Patients gain confidence in dealing with their issues. They learn how to change their behavior.

be perfect all the time. People would
still accept him for who he was. The
psychologist helped him worry less about
others' opinions. Many patients learn
techniques in therapy. These techniques
can be used in their daily lives.

MEDICATION IS A TEAM EFFORT

Medications can be helpful as well.
Prescribing the right ones can be tricky.
Some teens have serious issues that
require more than one prescription. Some
teens have risk factors. These factors can
include other health issues, or a family
history of substance addiction. These risk
factors can affect the medications that a
doctor prescribes.

A teen might have more than one mental disorder. But only one may be diagnosed. It is important for a doctor to get as much information about a patient

Teens can work with doctors to find the right medication.

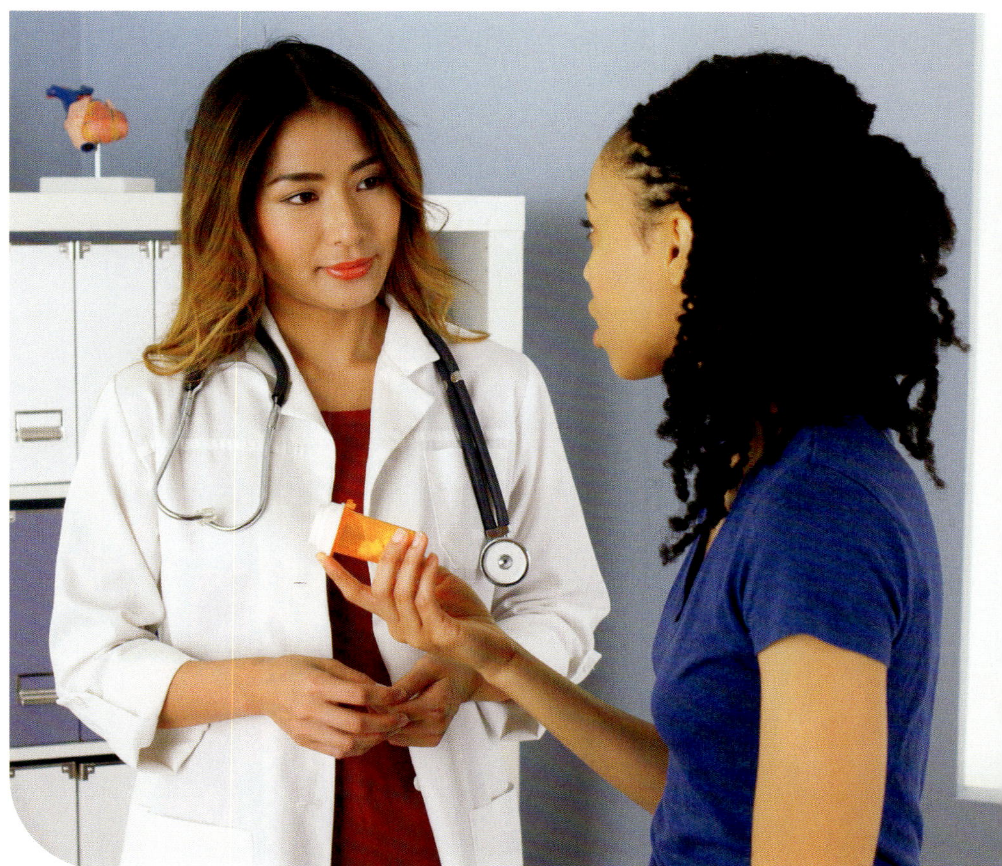

as possible before deciding to prescribe
a new medication. Powerful medications
come with some risks. A small percentage
of teens react badly to antidepressants.
Changing dosages or stopping a
medication abruptly can cause suicidal
thoughts in some patients.

Medications can affect patients
differently. Some teens suffer very few
side effects. Others have a harder time.
Hannah suffers from anxiety. She was
prescribed different drugs as a teen.
She talked to Young Minds, a mental
health organization. "Over the years, I've
tried more different types of medication than
I can count," she explained. "All . . . with
different benefits and strengths. . . . Some
had unpleasant side effects, a few seemed

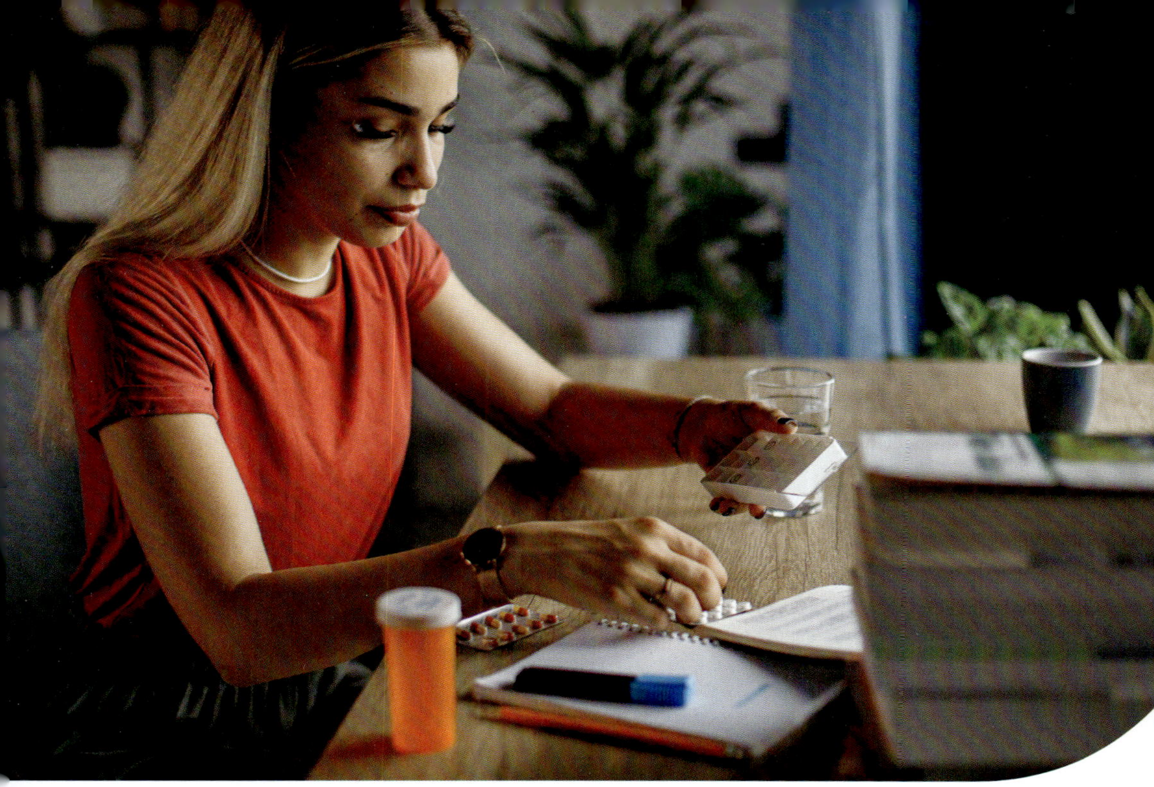

Prescribed medication should be taken as directed. Teens can use a pill organizer to keep track of their medication.

to make things much worse, and others had no impact whatsoever."[6]

Looking back, Hannah admits she quit certain medications if they did not work immediately. She would also not take them regularly. The first prescription she took was for Prozac. Years later, she returned to the drug and it finally worked. It kept

WHAT DOES SELF-CARE LOOK LIKE?

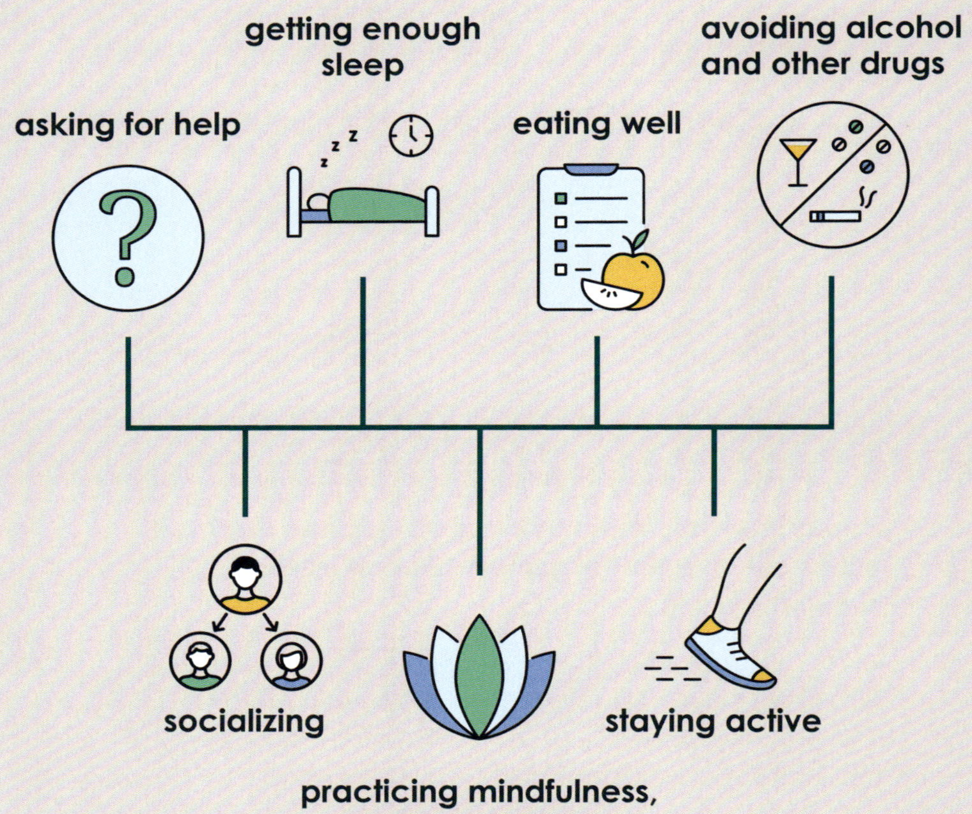

Speak with a health care specialist if mental health does not improve.

Practicing self-care can help improve overall mental wellness.

her emotions in check. It also reduced her
anxiety. Hannah says that sometimes a
person must try different things to find the
right treatment.

SELF-CARE AND OTHER TOOLS

Josephine, a 16-year-old from California,
has depression and anxiety. She says
therapy is not the only way to work through
one's issues on a day-to-day basis.
Practicing positive habits can also help.
These can be rituals and tasks that provide
comfort. They can be simple things such as
breathing exercises.

Some teens write down their feelings
by journaling. Creating art also lets them
express feelings that are hard to share.
Exercise routines can help to relieve stress.

Yoga and meditation can help teens focus on their breathing practices. For Josephine, self-care means something as simple as a skin care and a makeup routine. Getting enough sleep and eating healthy foods also helps her. Josephine's practices help her to feel safe. Josephine tells *California Globe*,

> ". . . therapy is important, but it took my family 2 years to find the right person. It is helpful for the times we talk, but what I personally realized I needed was also a day-to-day tool—something to do between sessions."[7]

FINDING A VOICE

In tenth grade, Kennedy had a serious anxiety attack. Her anxiety disorder is

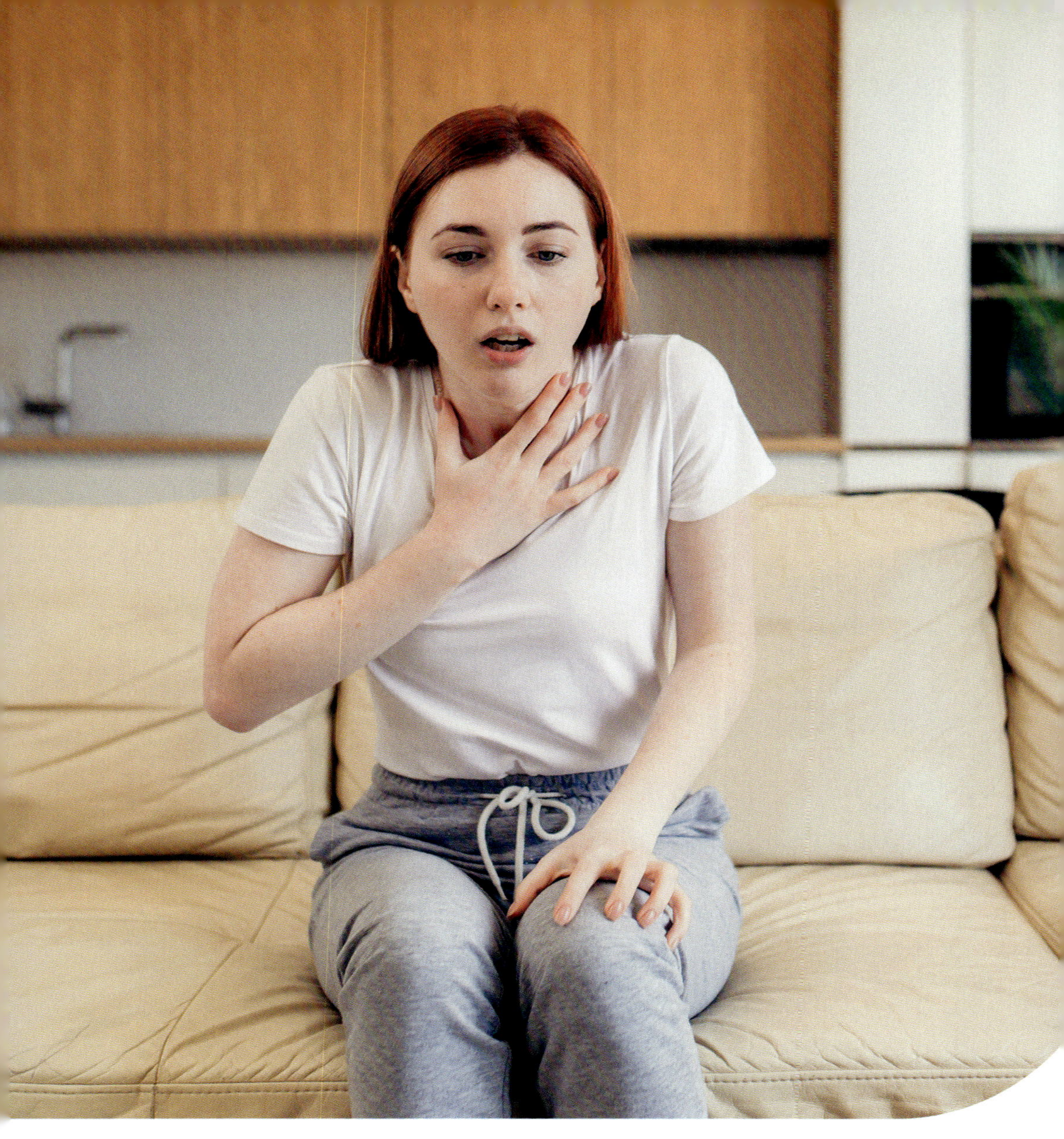

Rapid breathing can be a symptom of an anxiety attack.

an uncommon one. She suffers from
selective mutism. Selective mutism made
it hard for her to speak. Those who have it

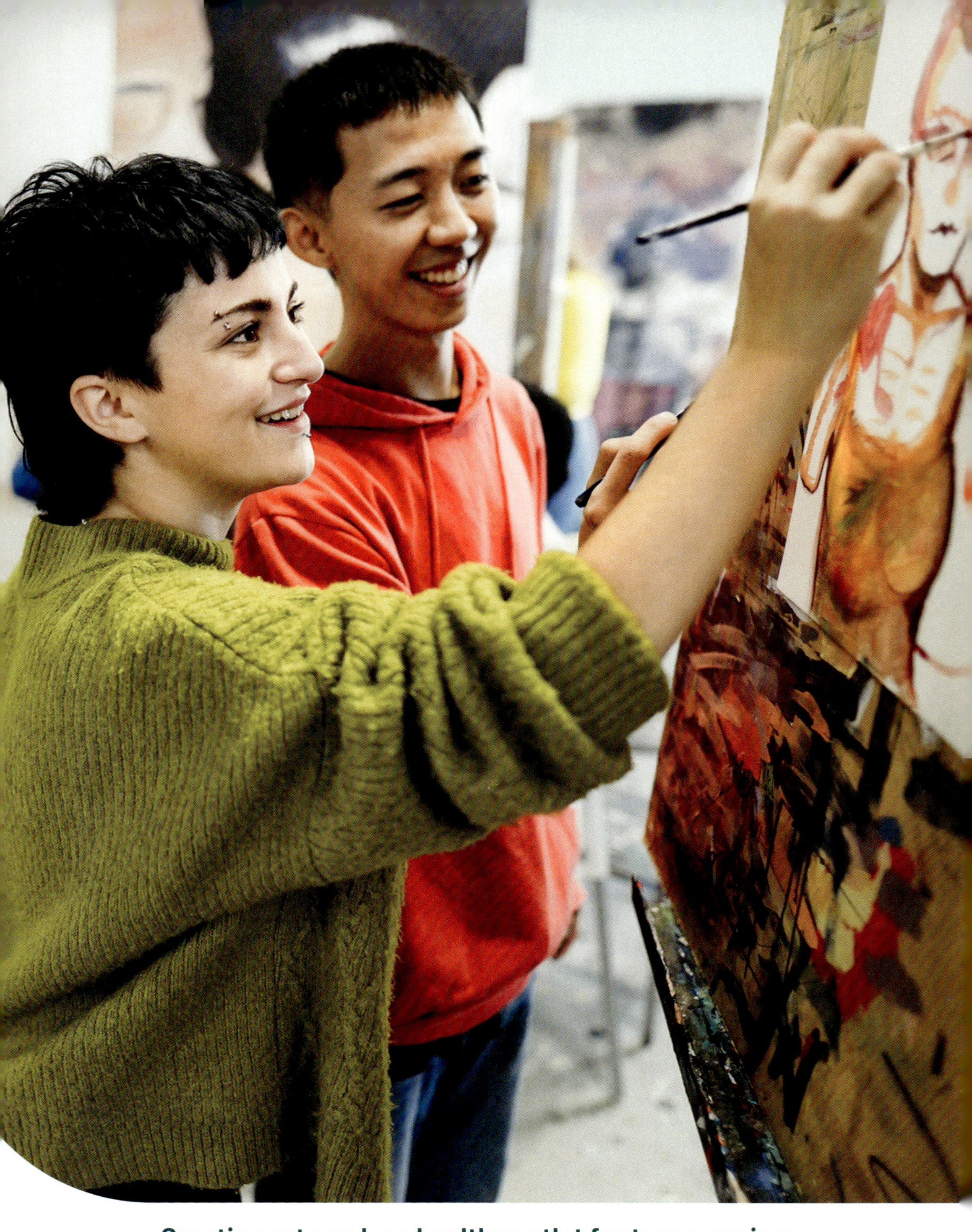

Creating art can be a healthy outlet for teens coping with mental illness.

often fear talking to anyone outside of close family members.

In 2019, Kennedy talked to CBS about her mutism. She said that as a 3-year-old, she did not speak to anyone in daycare for 6 months. Most people just thought she was shy. Her grandmother taught Kennedy her first song when she was 4 years old. As a teen, she found that singing made her anxiety go away. Dancing and creating art were also helpful outlets.

Kennedy wanted to share the techniques that had helped her. She started Arts for Anxiety in 2018. The programs help people express themselves through the arts. Kennedy's work includes performing for kids and veterans with PTSD.

REACHING OUT AND MOVING FORWARD

Socializing can also help teens cope with their mental illness. Studies show that teens who have social support tend to have better mental and physical wellness. Socializing can happen at school as well as at home.

Self-care routines, hobbies, sports, and other activities can also help. Teens can even form a mental health and wellness club in their own schools. Hope Squad, for example, is a suicide prevention program. It has chapters in more than 1,600 schools in the United States and Canada. Its mission is to help young people learn how to support and care for each other. Hope Squad teaches teens to look for warning signs in their friends.

Support exists in many forms. A strong support network and the right tools can provide lifelong benefits for mental well-being. A brighter future is always possible. Teens do not have to struggle with mental illness alone. Asking for help is the first step toward healing.

Those with mental illness may find support by spending more time with family.

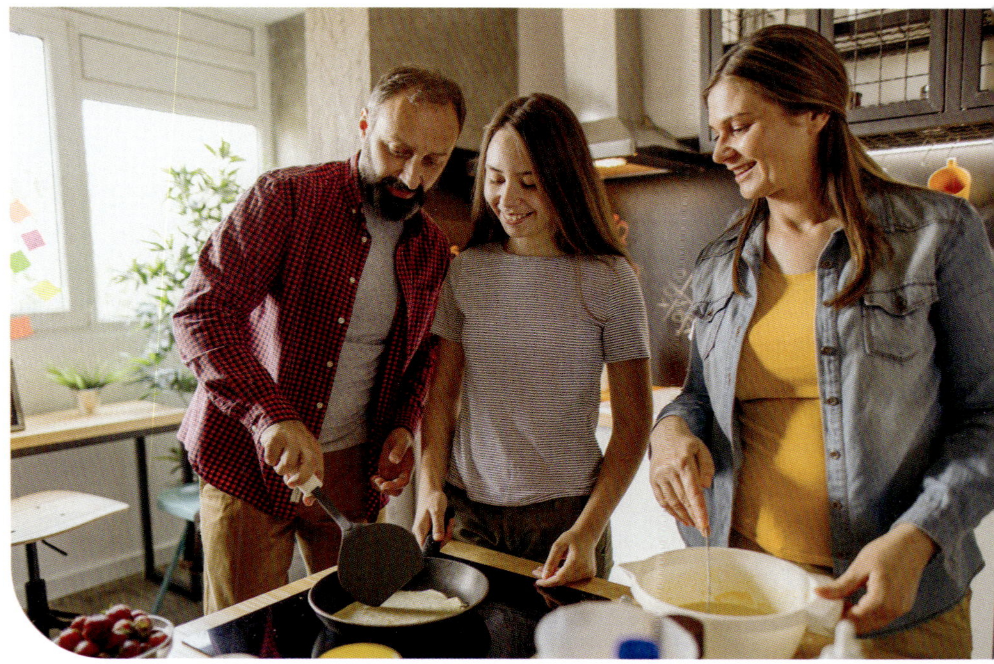

delusions

thoughts or beliefs that are not grounded in reality, and which are a symptom of serious mental disorders

diagnosed

when a medical or mental health professional decides the likely cause of symptoms a patient is experiencing

hyperactivity

the state of being more active than is appropriate for a particular time, place, or situation

impulsive

prone to taking action without thinking about the consequences

manic

having large feelings of excitement or energy above the typical amount, which can be difficult to manage

psychosis

a mental health symptom in which the mind loses connection with reality

purging

getting rid of something all at once

stigma

negative views that people hold against others who are seen as different

SOURCE NOTES

CHAPTER ONE: FEELING INTENSE EMOTIONS

1. Quoted in Craig Sawchuk, "What Is Depression? A Mayo Clinic Expert Explains," *Mayo Clinic*, October 10, 2022. www.mayoclinic.org.

CHAPTER TWO: OVERCOMING HURDLES

2. Quoted in Emily Matesic, "WI Teen Suicide Survivor Shares Recovery on TikTok," *ABC 7 Chicago*, April 3, 2021. www.abc7chicago.com.

3. Quoted in Jerry Bubrick, "First Person: A 13-Year-Old Learns to Fight OCD," *Child Mind Institute*, February 8, 2023. www.childmind.org.

4. Quoted in Deb Balzer, "Mayo Clinic Minute: How to Know If Your Teen Needs Mental Health Support," *Mayo Clinic News Network*, May 24, 2022. www.newsnetwork.mayoclinic.org.

CHAPTER THREE: LIVING WITH MENTAL ILLNESS

5. Quoted in Tobias J. Atkins, "My Lifelong Struggle with Social Anxiety," *Anxiety & Depression Association of America*, September 7, 2016. www.adaa.org.

6. Quoted in Hannah, "The Benefits of Changing My Mind-set When Taking Medication," *YoungMinds*, April 3, 2023. www.youngminds.org.uk.

7. Quoted in Josephine Urbon, "Putting a Face on Mental Health," *California Globe*, May 17, 2023. www.californiaglobe.com.

FOR FURTHER RESEARCH

BOOKS

Robin Bauser, *Social Media Anxiety.* New York, NY: Rosen, 2023.

Regine Galanti, *Anxiety Relief for Teens: Essential CBT Skills and Self-Care Practices to Overcome Anxiety and Stress.* New York, NY: Zeitgeist, 2020.

James Roland, *Teen Guide to Managing Mental Health.* San Diego, CA: ReferencePoint Press, 2024.

INTERNET SOURCES

A.W. Geiger and Leslie Davis, "A Growing Number of American Teenagers—Particularly Girls—Are Facing Depression," Pew Research Center, July 12, 2019. www.pewresearch.org.

Rory Linnane, "Milwaukee-Area Students Share Stories About Mental Health Challenges," *Milwaukee Journal Sentinel,* May 3, 2018. www.jsonline.com.

Sara Moniuszko, "Teen Mental Health Is in Crisis, Study Shows. What Can Parents Do?" CBS News, March 6, 2023. www.cbsnews.com.

WEBSITES

Alana Faith Chen Foundation
www.alanafaithchen.org

The Alana Faith Chen Foundation is a nonprofit organization that aims to raise funds for queer young people who are at risk of suicide. Funds raised go toward mental health treatment and therapy. Resources are available on their website.

National Alliance on Mental Illness (NAMI)
www.nami.org

The National Alliance on Mental Illness (NAMI) is a nonprofit organization that advocates for education, public awareness, and legislation surrounding mental health care.

The Substance Abuse and Mental Health Services Administration (SAMHSA)
www.samhsa.gov

The Substance Abuse and Mental Health Services Administration (SAMHSA) is part of the US Department of Health and Human Services (HHS). It is the main US government body in charge of national efforts to improve mental health treatment and education.

INDEX

IMAGE CREDITS

Cover: © Prostock-Studio/Shutterstock Images
5: © GagliardiPhotography/Shutterstock Images
7: © Monkey Business Images/Shutterstock Images
9: © F01 Photo/Shutterstock Images
11: © Eduard Figueres/iStockphoto
12: © fizkes/Shutterstock Images
14: © Pressmaster/Shutterstock Images
17: © Monkey Business Images/Shutterstock Images
18: © shironosov/iStockphoto
21: © Alex_Maryna/Shutterstock Images
22: © PeopleImages.com-Yuri A/Shutterstock Images
25: © Brian/iStockphoto
27: © Dima Berlin/iStockphoto
28: © Tory Zubovich/Shutterstock Images
31: © VH-Studio/Shutterstock Images
32: © VH-Studio/Shutterstock Images
35: © AnnaStills/iStockphoto
38: © Monkey Business Images/Shutterstock Images
41: © Africa Studio/Shutterstock Images
43: © pics five/Shutterstock Images
44: © AHPhotoswpg/iStockphoto
47: © Rocketclips, Inc./Shutterstock Images
49: © fotostorm/iStockphoto
50: © limeart/iStockphoto
53: © voronaman/Shutterstock Images
54: © DisobeyArt/iStockphoto
57: © mixetto/iStockphoto

Philip Wolny is a writer, editor, and copy editor hailing originally from Bydgoszcz, Poland. After growing up in the New York City boroughs of Queens and Brooklyn, he has since settled in Central Florida, where he resides with his wife and daughter.